Also by Dr. Stenbeck

Available from the usual on-line source

Books
Healing Yourself -- The Holistic Approach
  [An introduction to Holistic Self-healing.]

Heal Yourself Right Now!
  *[The Seven Priority Organ Levels for
  effective Nutritional/Holistic Treatment of
  all organs.]*

The 22 Unique Body Types
  (for Health and Weight Loss)

Q & A to Identify Your Body Type (Booklet)
  [Individual Type booklets are also available

Booklets
(Step-by-step instructions on healing yourself)

  #1 Start Healing with Positive Thinking
  #2 Mastering Positive Feelings for Health!
  #3 Spiritual Balance and Your Healing

The Sillevitic Body Type

Representing one of the 22 Body Types first described by Victor Rocine around 1900

The Rod Stewart, Carol Burnett Celebrity Body Type

For Kaye,
there at the beginning with Doc Severn,
and for Liberty,
continuing the holistic healing journey…

Disclaimer

About the Author

Educated in New Zealand and in the U.S.A., Dr. Stenbeck attained B.Sc. (NZ), M.S., and D.C. degrees. His holistic healing methods have been profiled in magazines (Esquire, McLean's, Playgirl, the Atlanta Constitution), and on TV in the USA and in Canada. He was the main contributor to the Warner Book, _The Eye/Body Connection_ by Jessica Maxwell that focused on the holistic healing relationships between the iris structure and organ genetics.

In the 1970-80's he was elected Fellow, Royal Society of Health, London; Fellow, American Association of Chemists; Member, American Association of Clinical Chemists; and Affiliate, Royal Society of Medicine, London. He studied naturopathy and Body Types with Dr. Bernard Jensen and Dr. Clifford Severn, and has practiced in medical partnerships where patients received the joint benefits of medical and holistic healing.

He is a member of Self-Realization Fellowship. To receive advice on any health issue from a holistic viewpoint, or to receive help with your body type, see his web site: *DrStenbeck.net*

———

Contents

* * *

The Sillevitic Body Type and Food Guide   1

* * *

The 22 Body Types:
Celebrity Examples

This Booklet contains the Sillevitic type. See <u>The 22 Unique Body Types</u> for all type descriptions.]

Thin Types

Atrophic   *Woody Allen / Audrey Hepburn*
       Stan Laurel / Calista Flockheart

Exesthesic   *Cher / Sarah Jessica Parker*
       (Female type only)

Marasmic   *President Obama / Princess Diana*
       James Stewart / Kate Blanchard

Neurogenic   *J.K. Simmons / Joan Rivers*
       Jon Cryer / Marin Hinle

Pathoferic   *(No celebrity males)*
       Blythe Danner / Gwyneth Paltrow

Sillevitic   *David Bowie / Shirley MacLaine*
       Rod Stewart / Carol Channing

Muscle Types

Calciferic	*Michael Jordan / Angelica Huston Abraham Lincoln / Grace Jones*
Carbogenic	*George Clooney / Lady Gaga Pres. G. Bush, Jr. / Meg Ryan*
Desmogenic	*Marlon Brando / Loni Anderson Daniel Craig / Tina Turner*
Eldic	*Ross Perot / Hillary Clinton Peter Falk / Sigourney Weaver*
Myogenic	*Pres. Bill Clinton / Sharon Stone Pres. John Kennedy / Julia Roberts*
Nervimotive	*Frank Sinatra / Elizabeth Taylor Mark Wahlberg / Natalie Wood*
Nitropheric	*Ben Affleck / Ava Gardner Kirk Douglas / Kate Winslet*
Pallinomic	*Pres. Donald Trump / Attorney General Janet Reno Bill O'Reilly (Fox) / Jane Russell*

Fat Types

Barotic   *Robin Williams / 'Mrs.Doubtfire'*
             Elton John / William Conrad

Carboferic   *Bill Murray / Roseanne*
             Billy Gardell / Melissa McCarthy

Hydripheric   *John Goodman / Shelly Winters*
             Wayne Knight / Jennifer Holliday

Isogenic   *Einstein / Oprah Winfrey*
             Phillip S .Hoffman / Queen Victoria

Lipopheric   *Rush Limbaugh / Rosie O'Donnell*
             Chris Christie / Camryn Manheim

Oxypheric   *Winston Churchill / Orsen Welles*
             Ella Fitzgerald / Gerry Spence

Pargenic   *Burt Reynolds / Katey Segal*
             Ron Perlman / Kirstey Alley

<u>Succinct Quote on Human Types</u>

From Victor Rocine, who first described discrete body types around 1900.

"A type is an order of people that differentiates and distinguishes itself by a general and similar form, brain-formation, chemistry, structure, build, immunity, tendencies, predisposition, resemblance, skin-pigment, and type characteristics based on observation and analogy.

"Or, in other words, people of a given type are similar physically and like-minded as if they were brothers and sisters—that is what type means.

"Everything in nature is made according to plan. Man only discovers that plan and gives it a name. The zoologist has not made the animals—he has only described the plan adopted by the wonderful Creator, and named the classes, sub-classes, etc.

"How important type research will be to humanity, time alone will make known."

———

Prologue

The esteemed scientist J. J. Berzelius, discoverer of several chemical elements, inspired Victor Rocine to research body types and to investigate the correlation between types and their diseases. Around 1890-1910, Rocine privately published his original findings on the mineral basis of different body types, and this present book exists because of his brilliant insights.

For many years, I studied with Dr. Clifford Severn who had been a personal student of Victor Rocine on body types, naturopathy, herbology, iris analysis, diet, and nutritional healing methods. He had a successful career as a lecturer and healer, and was one of those rare athletes with complete muscle control over his body. I saw him under a spotlight at 85 years of age, contracting and rippling every individual muscle in his perfectly developed body. Field-Marshal Jan Smuts, the WWII South African Prime Minister, devoted a full chapter of his autobiography to how Severn's healing methods had saved his life. In the 1950's, *Life* magazine did a four-page spread on Severn and his family. Fame he had.

Another Rocine student I studied with, Dr. Bernard Jensen wrote of Rocine's body type research and nutritional methods in his privately published book *The Chemistry of Man*.

This book is deeply rooted in Rocine's original work, and with that of Herbert Shelton, M.D., Ph.D. (at Harvard University in the 1930's). I integrated their research with newer dietary and nervous system data along with celebrity examples of each type, hopefully, making this material easier to digest and more entertaining for the reader.

Gayelord Hauser, another Rocine student I knew, was a celebrated health book author. He wrote a popular book on Rocine's types in the 1940's, *Types and Temperaments;* reputedly, he also introduced yogurt to the western world.

This book exists because of Rocine's creative brilliance and original discoveries in natural healing.

► *Rocine: "The soul creates the body type."*

Rocine taught that the soul chooses a body type and brain to live in, thus presenting different experiences and life lessons to master. Why were *you* born the way you are?

That is something to think about, especially if it is true! What would your soul purpose be to live in a particular body type. I provide some thoughts on this issue in each type description and try to assess from my experience with your type the particular lessons of life presented therein.

Rocine was as brilliant in his way as an Abraham Lincoln, Michael Jordan, Michael Phelps, Tony Robbins, or a Daniel Day Lewis—all *calciferic* types—rare, leaders, innovative, brilliant, and highly intelligent in their different fields of endeavor.

Celebrity examples exist for most types, not a duplicate of you, but someone who has your essence in their body-mind individuality. Knowing your type allows you to become a better you!

The celebrity examples provide further help in identifying your body type.

▶ *Rocine's classic findings are the backbone of this book. Integrated with Sheldon's research and with other dietary and food issues including mental, emotional, and spiritual attributes,*

Many people take nutritional supplements and try different diets without a doctor's advice. If this is your choice, use common sense, listen to body responses, and discontinue any allergic reactions to foods or nutritional substances.

———

The Sillevitic Body Type

* * *

"You may also have a physical or psychological feature not representative of your type such as height, weight, appearance, talent, weakness, strength, etc., due to biochemical errors, environmental influences, racial or cultural differences, and congenital or genetic issues. Nevertheless, the type identification of the average person is usually clear."

— *Victor Rocine*

Sillevitic Type
Celebrity Examples

If you think this is your type, be sure to look at **on-line photographs** *of these examples. Look for general similarities to yourself. Note that sub-types cause the differences in appearance between members of the same type. There are few celebrity examples of this rare type.*

ACTING

Billy Bob Thornton   Edward Fox
Matt Smith ("Crown" and "Dr. Who")
John Hurt   Adrien Brody

Carol Channing
Florence Henderson
Carol Burnett
Kristen Scott Thomas

VOICE

David Bowie   Rod Stewart
Beck

SPORTS

Dwight Stones (USA Olympic high jump)

RELIGION

Terry Cole-Whitaker (evangelist, author)

ARTS

Michael Tilson Thomas (conductor)
Doug Henning (magician)
Judith Cameron (author)

[Note: I personally knew one of these celebrities, and numerous other sillevitic people; once you know such a person you never forget them!]

Read the types and if still confused, you may choose to use the personal request for type identification from my web site *DrStenbeck.net*

———

Sillevitic Type Questionnaire

These questions describe the generic type, and not specifically you! If any question ever applied to you, then choose the True answer!

For Question 1 only:

A = True	B = Maybe	C = Untrue
15 points	7 points	1 point

1. Physically identify with celebrity example _____

Then...

A = True	B = Maybe	C = Untrue
5 points	3 points	1 point

---

2. Height is close to:
   Males: 5'7-6'2   Females: 5'5-5'9   _____
3. Usual weight is close to:
   Males: 130-170   Females: 125-155   _____
4. Slender body, weight easily controlled _____
5. Small, compact, strong muscles   _____
6. Always talking, talk with anyone   _____
7. Honestly express strong opinions
   (can sell anything)   _____
8. Hair lovely, fine, fair or dark   _____
9. Prominent cheek bones, with
   sunken cheeks   _____
10. High self-confidence, value, image   _____

11 Skin soft, thin, sensitive, often pale, attractive if healthy _____

12. Males have a long head, front to back, high crown, particularly in males _____

13. Slight facial hair in males; full head of hair is common _____

14. Long face from forehead to chin; females may have waxy rosy cheeks _____

15. Feel superior around peers _____

16. Sensitive lungs (or had lung disease) _____

17. Self-centered, often critical of others _____

18. Idealistic to help ecology, mankind _____

19. Excellent ability to socialize and converse with anyone (from homeless to Presidents!) _____

20. Are youthful looking _____

21. Happy, outgoing, eternally optimistic _____

22. May desire or crave coffee, sugar, nicotine, or alcohol _____

23. Strong ego, natural assertiveness or aggression may upset others; will confront anyone, anytime _____

24. Enjoy public speaking, teaching, influencing others _____

25. Often interested in new age healing, yoga and metaphysics _____

26. Pretty, attractive, handsome, ageless _____

27. Angular body frame, strong muscles, agility of dancers or gymnasts _____

28. Lean, bony, longer and thinner nose than average (especially males) _____

29. Cluttered home, office, car is typical _____

30. May suffer from excessive
    self-importance _____
31. Usually have prominent cheek-bones _____
32. Mouth often smaller, slightly terse lips _____
33. Voice jumpy, excited, friendly, happy,
    can talk forever! _____
34. Sunken chest; small or moderate bust _____
35. Will not compromise values or ethics _____
36. Malformed, fragile, irregularly-shaped
    teeth are common _____
37. Bony, muscular, strong back;
    shoulders bony, rounded _____
38. Narrow abdomen, hips; little fat (if
    healthy); long trunk _____
39. Charming, eloquent, sociable _____
40. Strong joints (if silicon intake is
    not excessive) _____
41. Assertive, or aggressive, rarely passive _____
42. "New age" interests: healing, yoga, etc. _____
43. Are able to communicate with anyone! _____
44. weakness in eyes, skin, or teeth _____
45. Have super-sales ability _____
46. May have unreal expectations about
    self and others _____
47. Difficult to stay in present time, or to
    keep dreams in reality _____
48. Kidney or bladder weakness _____
49. Unusual qualities and behaviors _____
50. Great procrastinators (may not
    walk the talk) _____
51. Usually disorganized or untidy _____
52. Often unrealistically optimistic _____

53. Weak skin or skin problems history   _____
54. Talent with voice, singing, sales, arts   _____
55. May have neurotic tendencies   _____
56. History or pain in bones, joints   _____
57. Humility is not a natural quality!   _____
58. Are definite risk takers   _____
59. Are exotic, unbending attitude   _____

Scoring

For question #1:

     A response: give 15 points   = _____
     B response: give 7 points   = _____
     C response: give 1 points   = _____

For questions #2—59:

     A response: give 5 points   = _____
     B response: give 3 points   = _____
     C response: give 1 point   = _____

     Total of the above points   = _____

Interpretation

   145—285:   **PROBABLY Sillevitic type**
   66—144:   POSSIBLY *Sillevitic type*
     <66:   NOT *Sillevitic type*

The Sillevitic Type

Rocine: "Sillevitic means 'light and easy.'"
Your body type utilizes more food <u>silicon</u>
than other types, and excessive intake
predisposes you to bone, joint, teeth, gum,
eye, skin, and connective tissue problems.

———

Y ou have a youthful appearance from childhood through old age with pretty, attractive, or handsome features. If healthy, you have lovely skin and a full head of attractive, blonde, or dark hair. Excessive silicon intake in childhood typically results in bad skin, teeth, and/or gums. If unhealthy, you should avoid silicon foods since you absorb them excessively; they are a major cause of your disease vulnerability. If healthy, you should minimize such foods!

▶ *Rocine: "You are like the lark—care-free, gay, and joyous."*

You are intelligent, creative, and extremely idealistic with high goals to accomplish for humanity. However, you achieve little if in your negative personality state—you may have a neurotic tendency. You are born to sell, to inspire people, and to sell any product.

You never give up. Your fervent belief in a cause induces others to follow you, but you may become bored and move on to more interesting projects.

▶ *You see your role as inspiring people to take action—not to nurture and keep them going!*

You age gracefully and maintain a youthful beauty; you are lean or gaunt when healthy, but always slender or slight. You may have nicotine addiction due to inherent lung weaknesses coupled with an excessively strong ego interfering with your lung balance. (Males who smoked are vulnerable to lung diseases.)

▶ *I knew several sillevitic males who smoked; one was a prior heroin and cigarette addict who stopped both "cold-turkey".*

———

Physical Similarity to Other Types

The *medeic* type (David Caruso, Madonna) is strong but often looks gaunt, plain, and worried.

The *neurogenic* type (J. K. Simmons, Joan Rivers) has a lean to medium build, with thinning hair.

The *atrophic* type (Woody Allen, Mia Farrow) is thin, and look fragile.

———

Average Height and Weight

| Males: | 5'7-6'2 | 130-170 | pounds |
| Females: | 5'5-5'10 | 125-155 pounds | |

You already know something about this type from their public persona and appearance, whether from seeing them yourself or from the celebrity examples. Blend such insights with the type descriptions and the types of your family and friends to discern their presence in your midst!

———

Sillevitic Type Description

The type description represents how you appear in everyday society. You may have a sub-type that alters parts of this description.

This type does not need youth drugs. You age gracefully and enviably. One *sillevitic* female I knew at age 85 looked about 50—she had to beat the old men on Viagra off with a stick! When young you have an angular body with small strong muscles and the agility of dancers or gymnasts. Most Olympian gymnasts, however, are *eldics, desmogenics, carbogenics, nervimotives, and myogenics.*

Head — A long head from front to back with a high crown in males is typical; females have a more proportional head.

Hair — You are fair or may have darker hair; when healthy your hair is soft, fine, and usually luxuriant and lovely. In some men, the hair is matted and oily.

Eyes — Mostly you have blue or brown eyes with thin fine eyebrows; you may have intense eyes with a large white sclera around the iris.

Ears — Your ears may be large (with an *eldic* sub-type).

Nose — A lean and bony nose, longer and thinner than average.

Face — You have a retreating forehead, a long face, with hollowed cheeks and prominent cheek-bones. The face holds little fat. The men may have only slight facial hair and have difficulty growing a full beard (as in the *atrophic and marasmic* types).

▶ *The female often shows rosy cheeks indicative of ill-health. This facial sign is different to the <u>atrophic</u> flush—your face may have a waxy appearance (from excessive silicon food intake).*

Mouth, Lips and Voice — The mouth and lips are often smaller, perhaps irregular in shape; your lips may be slightly terse. You have the gift of the gab and may talk for hours with a happy, excited, friendly, and optimistic voice!

Teeth — Many of you need cosmetic dentistry to correct dental weaknesses and malformations. Rarely, with a calcium sub-type, and with healthy silicon and calcium metabolism, you may have perfect teeth. You tend to cavities and irregular teeth due to silicon and calcium imbalances.

Skin — Your skin is soft, thin, sensitive, fragile, often white, and young looking. You usually age gracefully.

Neck — You have a thin neck with prominent muscles.

Muscles — Your muscles, ligaments, and tendons are soft, small, strong, moderately flexible, and easily strained. You enjoy aerobics, running, gymnastics, tennis, dancing, etc., and healthy outdoor activities. If unable to exercise because of pain, you probably already have distressed blood vessels, bones, joints, skin, teeth, eyes, or other connective tissue problems due to silicon excess and calcium metabolism problems.

Chest — A narrow and weak chest is characteristic; you usually have a small to moderate-sized bust, tending to lymph and breast congestion that heals with lymph massage, nutrition, and emotional releasing. Like the *atrophic and marasmic* types, you are vulnerable to childhood calcium disorders that distort your rib-cage.

Back and Shoulders — A bony, muscular, and strong back with rounded shoulders is common.

Hips and Abdomen — A narrow abdomen and hips with little excess fat is usual, if healthy. The trunk is long.

Arms and Legs — You have thin extremities of average or longer length.

Joints — Your abnormal silicon or calcium metabolism precludes you having strong joints and ligaments.

———

Sillevitic Personality Traits

If you are this type many, but not all, of the following characteristics are present—you may have overcome or moderated the negatives, but recognize that you once had several of them.

Positive Qualities

You may have many of the following traits:

- May have a super-sales ability
- Have high self: image, confidence, idealism
- Are not self-conscious: readily raise your voice
- Have unreal expectations about self and others
- Excellent oratory, speaking, convincing abilities
- Are very industrious, lively, friendly, enthusiastic
- Naturally assertive (some are aggressive and selfish)

▶ *You are excellent communicators, friendly and comfortable with kings or paupers. I have known you to function in high society with the greatest of ease, maintaining a happy, smiling, and comfortable demeanor, even if broke or unemployed.*

- Charming, eloquent, sociable, honest, noble, ethical
- Exotic, exclusive, egocentric, unbending, and friendly
- A powerful idealism and desire to help and inspire mankind
- Females easily hurt, may cry readily; have secretive feelings and difficulty in sharing emotional pain
- Friendly, relate to anyone, give people the benefit of the doubt (and thereby are easily hurt)

Potential Challenges

You may have evolved from, or not experienced these general faults, so do not dwell on them.

▶ *Rocine: "Things clutter up around you; a loving mate may help you become tidier!"*

I know several silicon people for whom this is true: you accumulate papers, magazines, books, and clothes and spread it around your homes, offices, and cars!

- Prone to fantasies and self-deceit
- Cannot keep dreams in realistic perspective

- Unlike several thin types, you are risk-takers
- May be critical, impulsive, egocentric, self-centered
- Humility is rarely present unless learned in childhood
- Changeable, adaptable, may be unduly familiar with people
- Some may leave the work-force and become destitute and homeless
- A disordered home and work environment is usual—you need a maid and an office manager [e.g., David Bowie was reported to be 'very messy'.]
- May discount other people's suggestions; may be poor bosses and managers; feel superior to others
- May have exotic, bizarre, exclusive qualities and behaviors that may confound others (and your doctors)
- Tend to internalize emotions of self: despair, longing, sorrow, sadness, or excessive ego in the heart and lungs
- Procrastination: you tend to postpone problem-solving (but believe that everything will work out okay if you wait long enough)
- Strong cravings or addiction to tobacco and/or coffee occurs in many of you,

because of self-negative lung emotions and an excessively strong ego

▶ *You tend to be egocentric, conceited or arrogant, and often suffer from a heightened sense of self-importance and aggrandizement; if female, this trait is threatening to many males. (You and the neurogenic type are vulnerable to neurotic tendencies: anxiety, compulsions, obsessions, depression, etc.*

———

Sillevitic Stress Management

You have vulnerable *mental* stress prevention because of your critical, impulsive, and egocentric beliefs; if people and systems do not align with your beliefs, you challenge everybody and authorities to follow your leadership—or someone will pay! You stress yourself through your beliefs and behaviors. This stress internalizes into your stomach, adrenals, and immune system creating seeds of ill-health. *Emotional* stress prevention is weak, and any of the above challenges may need your reprogramming help. *[If needing help managing these stresses, see my prior books.]*

———

Love

You usually attract practical mental types like the *carbogenic, carboferic, hydripheric, oxypheric, lipopheric, myogenic, and pallinomic.* There is a need for privacy and solitude for reading, writing, studying and meditating, etc. You tend to be insecure about the survival of your love relationship.

The males are not romantic lovers: you do what is required and then hurry back to your work; the females have a weak to moderate sexual drive, craving love, affection, and acceptance more than overt sex.

▶ *Rocine: "You manifest a playful, exhilarating intimacy, almost like an innocent child."*

Sillevitic Talents and Vocations

Abilities - *Artistic, acting, singing, healing, sales, the arts*

Your talents are in the arts and in inspiring and teaching others. You typically have difficulty working in successive approximations: set lower goals for yourself. You work effectively in the creative arts as artists, singers, actors, speakers, etc., or as a teacher of yoga, exercise, healing, nutrition, metaphysics, etc.

► *Your mind turns on at the prospect of communing, talking, and influencing people; in this sense, you are a social butterfly (opposite to the pathoferic type).*

The type information cannot predict what or who you will become, but you are capable of bringing a creative excellence or brilliance to whatever you do in life.

► *I have known, or observed you as drugless healers, psychologists, singers, architects, secretaries, teachers of yoga and dancing—and one heroin addict.*

Inabilities - *Organization, politics, science*

You are rarely found in medicine, science, mathematics, electronics, or engineering. Your mind is too scattered for straight-line thinking due to a active right brain! Encourage these children in public speaking, music, singing, acting, holistic healing, the creative and intuitive arts, etc.

———

Health Problems

When sick, you commonly experience health problems or diseases in any of the following tissues (due to internalized mental and emotional stress, and from excessive silicon intake):

Joints, Skin, Teeth, Gums, Skin, Eyes, etc. — These tissues are all very vulnerable to health problems. Nutritional supplements and emotional releases area needed to resolve such issues.

Lungs — The lungs are particularly vulnerable to disease and infection, due to self-sorrow, self-sadness, or self-ego imbalance superimposed on genetic lung weakness.

Lymph, Breasts — Congestion of lymph vessels is common, especially in the breasts, requiring nutrition, lymph drainage, and emotional releasing to prevent disease.

Arteries, Veins — These tissues are liable to disease.

Eyes, Ears, Sinuses — There is vulnerability to ear or eye diseases, or partial blindness (due to excessive silicon intake).

Gastro-Intestinal — Indigestion, swelling, malabsorption, and constipation problems are common (often because of mental stress and unresolved negative emotions locked in these organs).

Kidneys, Bladder — There is a urinary infection tendency in females.

Sexual Organs — Ovaries, uterus, breast, testes, and prostate problems are relatively common.

———

Sillevitic Acid/Alkaline Factor

[See Chapter 3 for details on this subject, along with the common symptoms found with people of different nervous system dominance.]

The genetics of your autonomic nervous system predispose you to needing a specific ratio of food acidity to alkalinity for your health and healing. You are born with an acid constitution, which means you need alkaline-ash foods for acid/alkaline balance. (Ash refers to the minerals left in your body after metabolizing foods.) Your nervous system genetics are *sympathetic* dominant, but because of a lifetime of eating excessive alkaline-ash foods, and from your nervous system vulnerability to becoming toxic, you need the intermediate Food guide. Eating silicon foods complicates your acid/alkaliane factor. If vegetarian, you need an **acid-ash** vegetarian diet.

> *For your healing, if in ill health or after about age 40-45, you need to aim for this approximate ratio of food selections:*
>   *50% Salads, vegetables, non-citrus fruits,*
>   *50% Proteins, carbohydrates*

▶ *Approximate your food ratios. On any particular day, it does not matter if one meal is mostly alkaline and another mostly acid—just try to balance it out for the day! If you make a mistake, try again tomorrow. It is a subjective call that you make, and what is done over time that makes the difference to your health.*

The Sillevitic Spiritual Factor

Skip this paragraph if uninterested in a philosophical perspective on your type!

▶ *Rocine: "The soul chooses the body type."*

If as souls, we choose the brain and body type to spend a lifetime in, it could be to learn certain spiritual lessons related to perfecting ourselves, and our humanity, in God's eyes.

What lessons does the type bring you? Only you can really decide what those lessons are. You know your weaknesses, faults, and behaviors towards others. You know things about yourself that Victor Rocine could never get from his research subjects when he first wrote about types. So search your mind for the answers.

Each discrete type has challenges of life lessons, spiritual goals, etc., and some of yours may be:

Faith — This is perhaps your most important challenge: you often feel separated from God (and have little faith). You need religion.

Excessive Idealism — You ache to right wrongs and to do something for mankind, the planet, the ecology: instead, just do what you can, and work on relaxing and taking care of yourself! The world will go on after you leave.

Egocentric, Arrogant, Aloof — Believe you are no better than anyone else in God's eyes! Yes, this is difficult for you to believe, but work on it; your loved ones and friends need your humanity, not your ego or and self-certainty that you are right about most things (which may be true).

Disorder — A disordered home and work environment interferes with your ability to plan, set goals, and to succeed: being tidy and organized improves your life quality.

▶ *Rocine: "You are quick to promise people help, or money, or almost anything, for you want people to be happy."*

————

A Sillevitic Story...

Bradley, 34, 6', lean and bony, had long limbs and a large mop of hair overlying his bright blue eyes. He complained of connective tissue problems: joint pains after exercising, skin, and respiratory infections.

Examination revealed no evidence of specific organ dysfunction, emotional or other stress problems to complicate his healing. His excessive vegetarian diet of alkaline-ash fruits, salads, and vegetables was the problem.

In addition he was eating excessive silicon foods: rice, seeds, nuts, strawberries, whole grains, and silicon herbs (oat straw, horse tail), which made him excessively alkaline. He avoided these foods, followed the type diet, and ate more *acid-ash* foods. He made a rapid recovery and maintained a pain-free condition.

————

Sillevitic Type
Mineral Food Needs

Apply this mineral data to the diet that follows the Thin type descriptions.

Excessive Foods:

- *Silicon*
- *Nitrogen (red meat)*
- *Alkaline-Ash citrus fruits, raw veges.*
- *Sulfur (cooked)*

Deficient Foods:

- *Magnesium*
- *Sulfur (raw)*
- *Nitrogen (vegetable)*
- *Acid-Ash vegetables, proteins (non-beef) and complex carbohydrates*

These deficient nutrients are common deficiencies in your type, and predispose you to ill-health.
If ill, be sure to use these lists with your <u>daily</u> food intake. If not ill, eat from the food lists 3-4 days <u>weekly</u> for health maintenance.
All food lists are in descending order of concentration and value to you; choose servings of foods in the upper half of each list first! One serving is ½ cup.

Sillevitic Excessive Foods -

Silicon is invariably excessive in your tissues, and avoiding such foods is essential for normal silicon metabolism and improved health. You absorb silicon at a greater rate than the average person, and often eat such foods excessively until diseased.

Nitrogen (red meat) should be eaten 0-1 times monthly.

Alkaline-ash citrus fruits and raw vegetables are usually excessive in your dietary selections; minimize such foods, and eat more daily acid-ash foods (proteins and carbohydrates).

Sulfur from <u>cooked</u> sulfur vegetables is contraindicated, because it brings excess sulfur acid toxicity into your tissues and may cause emotional instability, vague aches, and pains. Avoid cooked sulfur foods: cauliflower, cabbage, rutabaga, garlic, spinach, carrot, and Brussels sprouts. Raw sulfur foods preclude this happening.

———

Deficient Foods -

If ill or diseased, it is important to correct these mineral deficiencies.

Magnesium is often deficient in your type, and is particularly important for your heart and digestive function.

Sulfur in *raw* form is deficient in your tissues (see above).

Nitrogen (vegetable, non-red meat) is needed; if not a dedicated vegetarian, be sure to eat good poultry, fish, or eggs, about 3-5 times weekly. If vegan or vegetarian be sure to have 25-30 grams of a protein drink daily (in addition to vegetarian sources).

Acid-ash vegetable proteins and carbo-hydrates are often deficient in your diet.

Note -

The following recommendations are for the generic type. Additionally, you may need from a holistic healer or nutritionist something more specific for your individuality.

Minimize
Excessive Foods

Silicon: *0-2 servings/week*

Seeds and nuts, herbs (Oat Straw, Horsetail), strawberries, whole rice, whole oats, apples, iceberg and Boston lettuce, peanuts, asparagus, barley, bran, cereals, breads, alfalfa, whole wheat, soybeans, curry powder, cabbage, dandelion greens, dried figs, cucumbers, onions, pumpkin, ripe olives, milk, most cheeses, peas, dark greens, kelp, lima beans, rye, onions. [Important: You usually over-eat these foods, making youe excessively alkaline—and sick!

Nitrogen (beef): *0-1 times/month*

Beef, red meats

Alkaline-Ash Foods: *0-2 servings/week*

Salads and raw vegetables (Avoid citrus fruits like orange, lemon, lime and their juices.)

Eat
Deficient Foods

Magnesium: *1-2 servings/day*
Kelp, parsley, blackstrap molasses, brewer's yeast, cashew, buckwheat, dried prunes, peanuts (dry roasted), peanut butter, baked potato (with skin), black-eyed peas (cooked), pinto beans (cooked), brown rice (cooked), baked beans.

Sulfur (raw): *1-2 servings/day*
Cauliflower, garlic, spinach, carrots, horseradish, almonds, coconut

Iodine: *1-2 servings/day*
Seaweed, kelp, fish, eggs, yogurt, Turkey breast, Navy beans

Acid-Ash Foods: *1-2 servings/day*
Cooked carbohydrate vegetables (yams, squash, potatoes, pumpkin, etc.), plums and cranberries; and proteins (below)

Nitrogen (non-red meat, vegetable):

Eggs, poultry, fish —3-5 times weekly
Legumes (peas, beans), pasta —as desired
Protein drink daily —if vegetarian

Note: Eat any healthy foods you desire, but be sure to include type foods in your daily choices.

Sillevitic Nutritional Supplements

- **Multi-Vitamins-Minerals -**
  [Take all supplements with food.]
  2 capsules daily containing 500 mg. calcium
  (with magnesium)/ twice daily
- **Lecithin** —
  About 1,300 mg/ three times weekly
- **Herbs** —
  Brain detox — Kyolic garlic or chamomile
  Organ detox — Golden Seal or Chickweed
  Mental balance — Chamomile
  (Take one capsule, twice daily, for one month;
  then one, three times weekly.)
- **Evening Primrose or**
  Flaxseed Oil —
  1 soft-gel/ day
- **Other** —
  Chlorophyll, blue-green algae, green
  magma, spirulina, alfalfa, or other source
  (Take as directed, three times weekly)

Note: Be sure to take these supplements if you
have ill-health. If you are in good health, take
them at least 3-4 times/week.

Important Sillevitic Health Concerns

▶ *If vegan or vegetarian have 25-30 grams of protein daily in a drink (and find a good doctor)! You require a variety of vegetarianism where you eat liberally of proteins and carbohydrates (an acid-ash diet).*

SILLEVITIC FOOD GUIDE

Aim for –

50% Proteins, complex carbohydrates
50% Fruits (non-citrus), raw vegetables
and
70% Cooked foods
30% Raw food diet
Avoid silicon foods!
Take the recommended supplements.

Eat Acid-Ash Foods

- *Proteins* like soybean, protein drinks, poultry, fish, or eggs
  (3-5 times weekly)

- *Complex carbohydrates* like yams, squash, potatoes, pumpkin, corn, lentils, peas, beans, green vegetables (3-5 times weekly)
- *Cooked vegetables:* as desired (except silicon vegetables)

Avoid

- *Silicon foods* (only 0-2 times <u>week</u>).
- *Natural grains, breads, cereals, nuts, seeds, citrus fruits* (0-2 times weekly); these foods bring in excessive silicon and alkalinity, with consequent ill-health and weight gain. The sickest silicon people are those on steamed grain and vegetable diets.

Sillevitic Weight Loss

Theoretically, being a *Thin* type, you require that Food Guide, but it is inappropriate because of your special needs. Stay with your type instructions and you will find the right way to eat for your health and weight loss.

Avoid all grains, breads…(as above).
Avoid all silicon foods.
Avoid all citrus fruits.
Avoid all simple sugars: white sugar,

brown sugar, high fructose corn syrup, honey, maple syrup, molasses, jellies, candy, ice-cream, fruit and soda drinks.

Notes

- *Gluten* sensitivity is common
- *Protein* drink, have daily, about 25-30 grams.
- *Eat* your body type deficient mineral foods daily.
- *Follow* your *Sillevitic Factors* (as above) food instructions.
- *Exercise*: your body type requires only light daily exercise (like yoga, walking, roller-skating, etc.).
- *Mental balance and positive thinking:* everyday life stresses you easily, causing adrenal hypoglycemia, low blood sugar; you need to take these supplements: *calcium/magnesium*, two capsules, twice daily with food; and *chamomile,* two capsules with food.
- *Hypoglycemia:* this hormonal imbalance stops fat loss, and usually initiates more fat production, so it is vital to deal with this problem: take *pantothenic acid,* 500 mg/twice daily with food (see my earlier books to resolve this problem).
- *Calories:* As with any dietary approach, calories in must be *less than* calories out!

Most markets sell a calorie booklet; make notes of your daily intake, and in most instances keep it under about 1500 calories/dav.

———

Thin Types
General Food Guide

(Vegetarian or Semi-Vegetarian)

Important Note

————

The Food Guide addresses the <u>Acid-Alkaline</u> aspect of your food intake, along with the <u>Type Mineral</u> factor presented throughout this book. It does <u>not</u> necessarily address calories or other dietary factors that may be pertinent to your personal health needs whether medical or appropriate for some other dietary need. So use your common sense and just include the factors described here with whatever healthy dietary choices you usually make.

For other nutrient information, consult with nutritional books or with holistic nutritional doctors. I particularly recommend the advice of Andrew Weil, M.D.

————

General Food Guide

This chapter presents a general Food Guide, upon which you superimpose the nutritional information from your type chapter.

———

Meat/Flesh Intake

Most muscle types should limit red meat to once or less weekly, while eggs, lamb, fish, or poultry are excellent in moderation. If ill or diseased, be sure to eat daily, one or two servings from each *deficient minerals* list. If not ill, eat them at least three times weekly for health maintenance. If this diet is similar to your present diet, but healing is sluggish, then:

- Decrease your carbohydrate and protein intake by about one-third
- Increase your fruit, salad, and vegetable intake by about one-third
- Consult with a holistic doctor, preferably one versed in nutritional and emotional evaluation

———

Over-Acid or Over-Alkaline?

Just as a log of wood burned in your fireplace leaves a mineral-ash, food ash refers to the minerals remaining after metabolizing foods in your tissues:

- Fruits, vegetables **alkalinize** tissues
- Proteins, carbohydrates **acidify** tissues

Usually You Are Over-Acid Due To:

- Excessive intake of dairy foods
- Excessive intake of proteins and carbohydrates
- Deficient intake of fruits, salads and vegetables
- Accumulated metabolic waste-acids (from years of eating excessive acid-ash foods, meats and carbohydrates, and from lack of exercise)
- You need to estimate the ratio of foods eaten. Generally, eat the following *approximate* ratios for your health:

50% <u>Alkaline-ash</u> foods *(fruits, salads, vegetables)*

50% <u>Acid-ash</u> foods *(complex carbohydrates like starches, grains, cereals, breads, flour products; and proteins)*

Approximate your food ratios. On any particular day, it does not matter if one meal is mostly alkaline, and another mostly acid—just try to balance it out for the day! If you get it wrong, try again tomorrow. It is a subjective call that you make, and it is what you do over weeks, months, or years that make the difference—not on any one or two days.

———

Important

- Minimize white sugar and alcohol intake.
- If desired, interchange lunches for dinners.
- Never eat foods you are allergic to, no matter what I recommend; if allergic, or suspect a food allergy, eliminate it and substitute from your type mineral lists.
- Eat the right foods 80-90% of the time and the Food Guide will work for you; unlike some types you do not have to live out of a health food store (although such foods are healthier for you).

▶ *Omit eating the excessive minerals in your type chapter, and be sure to eat one or two servings from the deficient list daily.*

On any particular day, it does not matter if one meal is mostly alkaline, and another mostly acid—just try to balance it out for the day! If you make a mistake, try again tomorrow. It is a subjective call that you make, and it is what you do over weeks, months, or years that make the difference—not on any one or two days or weeks.

———

Acid/Alkaline Genetics, Dietary-Ash, and Raw Food Needs

This chart shows the Rocine types, their acid or alkaline food needs, and the percentage of raw foods needed for your health and healing.

- Apply your Type Minerals to the Food Guide

Type Genetics	Acid/Alkaline Genetics	% Food-Ash Needed	% Raw Food
Atrophic	Acid	80% alkaline	90
Exesthesic	Acid	70% alkaline	70
Marasmic	Acid	70% alkaline	50
Neurogenic	Acid	70% alkaline	50
Pathoferic	Alkaline	50% alkaline	30
Sillevitic	Alkaline	50% alkaline	30

The above percentages vary depending on aging and the health of individual types.

▶ *Observe the excessive minerals in your type chapter, and be sure to eat one or two servings from the deficient list daily (or, several times weekly).*

Important

- Minimize white sugar and alcohol intake.
- If desired, interchange lunches for dinners.
- Never eat foods you are allergic to no matter what is recommended; if allergic or suspect a food allergy, eliminate it and substitute from your type mineral lists.
- Eat the right foods 80-90% of the time and the *Food Guide* will work for you.
- You may have allergies to wheat, corn, other grains, sugar, alcohol, and milk (examine your body reactions to these foods for fatigue, sinusitis, joint pain, skin rash, and gastro-intestinal reactions). Note that the *atrophic* type *requires* dairy foods for health and healing.
- Living out of a health food store is unnecessary (although such foods are healthier for you). If you want dietary perfection in your healing efforts, eat organic foods (from a health food store).

General Food Guide

[Superimpose the nutritional information from your Type Chapter into this Food Guide.]

Breakfast

FRUIT *salad, fresh (with citrus fruit) and* *protein: yogurt, kefir, milk, cheeses, or raw seeds or nuts* — *3+ times/week; or*

CEREALS *(whole grain), fruit, seeds, and nuts as desired* — *2+ times/week; or*

EGGS *(1-2) with lettuce, tomato, veges, non-wheat toast* — *0-3 times/week; or*

OTHER *choices* — *0-1 times/week*

Daily Liquids

Coffee, teas — *0-1 cups*
Pure water, citrus, fruit, or vegetable juices, soups, other — *as desired*
Wheat is a common allergy: avoid white breads; eat sour dough, millet, or oat breads instead.
Note: For in-between snacks, have fruit or vegetables, with seeds or nuts.

Lunch

SALADS, mixed green, with <u>protein</u> (cheese, soy, seeds, egg, etc.) Dressing: virgin olive oil and vinegar, low-fat dressings — 3-5 times weekly; and/or

VEGETABLES with salad (and a <u>protein</u>: yogurt, cottage cheese...) — 1-3 times/week; or

FRUIT salad (like breakfast)
   — 1-2 times/week; or

SANDWICH, whole grains, cheese and /or other non-flesh <u>protein</u>; small salad
   — 0-2 times/week; or

OTHER choices
   — 0-1 times/week

* Other oils less ideal; soybean oil is a common allergen; minimize commercial dressings.

Dinner

VEGETARIAN meals: include legumes, tofu, cheese, cottage cheese, seeds, nuts, egg, etc. (and/or salad) — 2+ times/week; or

POULTRY/FISH (3-6 oz.), salad and/or vegetables — 0-2 times/week; or

WHOLE GRAIN PASTA, cooked (barley, rice, millet, etc.), and salad/or vegetables — 0-2 times/week; or

OTHER choices — 1-2 times weekly

DESSERTS: Fruits, fresh or low-sugar desserts — as desired

Note: Be sure to include one or more selections from your type food lists in your daily food intake.

Note. If *vegetarian,* substitute flesh proteins with seeds, nuts, legumes, and other vegetables. You are vulnerable to being protein deficient so be careful to eat sufficient proteins and/or include a daily protein drink!

Food Guide Notes

Steamed Vegetables — Minerals are lost in the boiling of vegetables, so steaming or wok cooking is best.

Food Combinations — Eating proteins at the same meal with starches often results in indigestion, gas or constipation (as does eating fruit and starch together). For those of you with weak digestive systems, watch how this or other inharmonious combinations may be affecting you.

Periodic Detox Dieting — If you over-indulge in acid-ash foods, you need occasional elimination diets for tissue waste-acid removal, supervised by a nutritional doctor.

Minimize —
- Plums, cranberries, and their juices
- Commercial, sugared, and fatty salad dressings
- Red meats, processed meats, wines, alcohol, and milk
- Coffee, white sugar, fructose, and chemical sugar substitutes
- Exposure to drugs, environmental chemicals, pesticides
- Avoid eating allergic foods

Healthy Weight — You have a good ability to lose and control weight by following the Food Guide instructions. If you gain weight, the most common reason is liver or kidney irritation due to food allergies or negative emotions—the key is to eat non-allergic foods. The *atrophic and marasmic* types usually need to gain weight. (Obviously, if you have a medical condition that contradicts this advice, do not change your diet!)

In addition to your body type needs, other holistic healing matters also need your attention. I strongly suggest that you refer to my web site and earlier books for that information: *DrStenbeck.net*

———

In Conclusion

It may be difficult to discern your type from the *neurogenic and atrophic* types, and the lean and strong *calciferic, nervimotive, and medeic* types. Study them well and you will see the diff-erences.

———

Appendix

Brief Extracts from
The 22 Unique Body Types

Appendix A

Types
(Brief extract)

Type comes from 'typus' meaning an image or impression, the study of types being called typology.

▶ *Rocine: "A combination of mental and structural features is consistently found in people of the same type."*

Rocine wrote that all types are a mixture of positive and negative qualities. He based his work on the biochemical individuality of our *mineral* absorption and utilization. Of course, all minerals are absorbed, but he postulated that different types of people *selectively* absorb certain minerals, to a greater or lesser extent, requiring specific mineral foods for their enhanced health and healing.

▶ *The type information cannot predict what or who you will become, or how successful or not, but your type is capable of bringing a creative excellence to whatever you do in life. If your type has negative qualities that you disagree with, remember that they are only tendencies and may or may not manifest in you.*

This book enlarges on Rocine's premise (early 1900's), integrated with the later research of Herbert Sheldon, M.D., Ph.D., at Harvard University (1930's), along with my fifty years of observations and experience with this subject.

Comparing your shared physical (and sometimes psychological) descriptions with the Celebrity Lists further assists the identification of your type. It is not that you will look exactly like, or be a twin to, any particular celebrity. Look closely at a celebrity's features: face, profile, height, weight, head, etc. If you know something about their talents, beliefs, success and failure spheres, health and weight challenges, attitudes and behaviors, etc., then you get clues as to what your type may be.

———

Understanding Types and Sub-Types

Each of us has a clearly discernible dominant type. Visualize the celebrity examples from movies, politics, sports, the arts and public life, and try to identify with their physical features. Look for similar features, remembering that you will not recognize all attributes in yourself. You are not looking for your twin!

The sub-type issue is the main reason people of the same major type can look so different. Remember that a type description does not characterize you exactly, but depicts your individual variant of a type.

▶ *The type questionnaire pinpoints the major features of that type: if the celebrity examples are unhelpful, you may be an unusual variant (in which case ignore the celebrity issue and give yourself 7 points on Question 1).*

———

Minerals

Minerals are essential life nutrients that accelerate enzyme and chemical reactions and provide a basis for your body typing. Although found in all tissues, different minerals tend to be concentrated in certain organs, their presence or absence contributing to the healing of such tissues; e.g., zinc accelerates prostate healing; calcium and manganese promote bone, joint and connective tissue healing.

Specific foods nurture each type, some people needing meats for their health others needing a vegetarian diet. A high potassium diet nurtures one person, while another needs high sulfur, calcium, zinc, or another mineral.

Mineral Digestion and Absorption

Compared to vitamins, minerals are *difficult* to digest, absorb, and utilize. In people with strong digestive systems, this aspect may not be important. The following factors should be in place for optimal mineral metabolism:

1. Stomach Hydrochloric Acid Production
2. Parathyroid Hormone Balance
3. Organ Toxic Metal and Chemical Removal
    [See details in The 22 Unique Body Types.]

––––––

Total Body Healing

Note that from a holistic healing perspective, in addition to minerals and type information, the following healing factors are necessary:

> *Nutrient Balance*
> *Mental Balance*
> *Emotional Balance*
> *Spiritual Balance*
> *Detoxifying Integrity*

The above factors are all important to your total healing especially if you are interested in self-healing (see my earlier books).

––––––

Appendix B

Researchers
(Brief extract)

The predominant workers in this area of human individuality from around 1880's to the 1960's are Herbert Sheldon, M.D., Ph.D., Roger Williams, Ph.D., and Victor Rocine, D.Sc.

Much information on Sheldon's research exists on-line and in medical psychology libraries; for interested readers there are other lines of research published in the last century. This present book is primarily about Rocine's body types.

Herbert Sheldon M.D., Ph.D.

In contrast to Rocine, Sheldon at Harvard University in the 1930's was trained in the scientific method and did painstaking research and publishing on human individuality. In comparing his findings with Rocine's work, a direct putative correlation is visible.

Roger J. Williams, Ph.D.

Another significant researcher in human individuality is the renowned scientist and biochemist, Roger J. Williams. He demonstrated that different people have varying levels of nutrients, enzymes, and other metabolic chemicals in their bloodstreams.

▶ *Williams's research firmly expands on the premise of individual nutritional needs in human beings. If interested in his research, I highly recommend his book Biochemial Individuality.*

Victor Rocine, D.Sc.

Note that when a negative feature is indicated, say neurotic tendencies, all members of the type are <u>not</u> that way; it is a type tendency reported by Rocine.

Rocine studied type-related diseases finding links between mineral and dietary factors with individual types and their diseases. In each body type, one or more dominant minerals are preferentially absorbed and utilized over other minerals.

He recognized discrete body types from their physical appearance finding genetically based mineral dominance to be the determining feature. He also correlated their physical features with psychological characteristics.

———

Appendix C

Genetics, Types, and Diet
(Brief extract)

This section deals with how nervous system genetics helps determine your eating choices for health: you are either born to be a predominant meat eater, a partial or complete vegetarian, or something between the two. The genetic factor determining this dietary aspect is the *sympathetic and parasympathetic* components of your central nervous system. This represents a basic factor in eating for health.

This chapter helps you understand your dietary inheritance, although instinctively, you may already have arrived there!

- If born **sympathetic** dominant you are *genetically acid*, desiring a predominantly *vegetarian* diet for your health (about 70% fruit, salad, vegetables to 30% proteins and carbohydrates).

- If born **parasympathetic** dominant you are *genetically alkaline*, desiring a predominantly *carnivorous* diet for your health (about 70% proteins, carbohydrates to 30% fruits, salads, vegetables). Few of you ever choose to become vegetarian because of the difficulty in satisfying your protein needs without meats.

- If born *intermediate* dominant you may eat food groups with little concern for the acid/alkaline factor. However, after age 40, you need a semi-vegetarian diet for healthy eating.

———

Chart of Relative Nervous System Dominance

In the following Chart, if you relate to many of the symptoms on one side you probably have that nervous system dominance; relating to both sides indicates *Intermediate* dominance.

If Vegetarian (Over-acid) --
Eat 70% fruits, salads, vegetables
And 30% proteins, carbohydrates

If Carnivore (Over-alkaline) --
Eat 70% proteins, carbohydrates
And 30% fruits, salads, vegetables

If Intermediate --
Eat 50:50 of acid and alkaline-ash foods

Make an *approximate* estimate of your daily acid and alkaline food intake (such ratios varying from type to type).

———

Symptoms of Relative Genetic Dominance

Vegetarians (Over-acid)	Carnivores (Over-alkaline)
Sympathetic Dominance	Parasympathetic Dominance
little or no flesh desire	desire flesh
easily constipated	rarely constipated
slow digestion	fast digestion
easily dehydrated	not dehydrated
strong thirst	low thirst
pale face	flushed face
high pulse after food	slow pulse after food
easy gag reflex	slow gag reflex
cool dry skin	moist warm skin
nervous stomach	calm stomach
little eyelid blinking	much blinking
nervous tendency	mostly calm
slower healing	faster healing
low oxygen-uptake	good oxygen-uptake
easily breathless	seldom breathless
insomnia common	sleep easier
few muscle cramps	some night cramps
calcium deposits rare	get calcium deposits

Appendix D

Help Identifying your Body Type with Dr. Stenbeck

If you desire help in identifying your body type, follow these instructions, and answer the questionnaire. For further information and fees, send me an email from page one of the website:

DrStenbeck.net

First name: _____

Country of birth: _____

Upload photos and send to the above website:

■ Head and shoulders: front and side views

■ Full body: front and side views

■ Also 1-2 teenage views

■ If possible, casual photos of mother, father, siblings

MY TYPE CLASS MAY BE: _____

(Thin, Muscle, or Fat)

AGE - _____

HEIGHT - _____ feet/inches

MY WEIGHT - _____ pounds

Heaviest at age: _____

- Lightest as adult: _____

- Estimate age 15: _____

VISION - Excellent Average   Poor:

HAIR -   Natural color: _____

- Thin/thick? _____

- balding? _____

SKIN - Quality: _____

- History of acne, boils, other:

_____

_____

TEETH   - Strong   Weak   Dentures

- Cavity history: Many   Moderate   Fev

MUSCLES - Strong   Average   Weak

Sports played _____

JOINTS   - Strong   Average   Weak

HEALTH - Childhood diseases?

_____

_____

- Adult diseases?

_____

AVERAGE DIET

- Beef _____ (times/week)

- Poultry _____ (times/week)

- Fish _____ (times/week)

- Eggs _____ (times/week)

- Water _____ (glasses/day):

- Vegetarian? Vegan? _____

- Other? _____

- Did your childhood diet differ? _____

The above will help me know who you are! I will send you a follow-up questionnaire for further help in identifying your body type.

Appendix E

On-line Health Consultation
with Dr. Stenbeck

For further information, or to comment on this book, or to receive a response on any health issue from a holistic viewpoint, send an email inquiry from page one of my website:

DrStenbeck.net

Following that, I will suggest further healing needs, which we may pursue with an on-line consult.

———

Appendix F

Notes

See my book *The 22 Unique Body Types,* available at the usual online source, for further information and details on all of the 22 Types. The Appendix in that book has further information about:

Mineral Functions and Food Sources

Further Reading